CW00351649

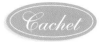

Fabulous Facials

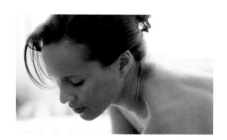

KUDOS

Published by Kudos, an imprint of Top That! Publishing plc.
Copyright © 2004 Top That! Publishing plc,
Tide Mill Way, Woodbridge, Suffolk, IP12 IAP, www.kudosbooks.com
Kudos is a Trademark of Top That! Publishing plc

Contents

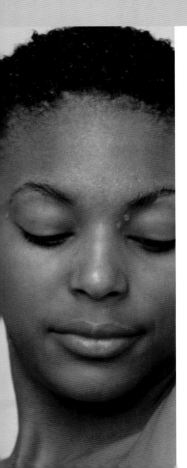

Introduction

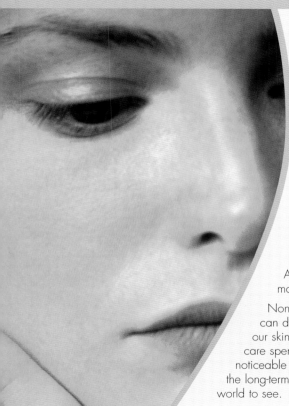

Long-term **benefits**

Making the most of the face we're born with is the aim of most women. Although we can't change our physical attributes, we can change the health and texture of our skin and learn to feel confident with our faces. Learning how to care for our skin through diet, cleansing and natural products and minor changes in lifestyle can have dramatic effects. Added to that the magic of make-up can work minor miracles.

None of us can stop time, but we can delay some of the effects it has on our skin. The rewards of a little time and care spent each day on our faces will be noticeable in only a very short time, and the long-term benefits will be there for all the world to see.

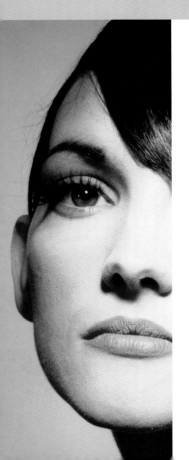

The word 'cosmetics' comes from the Greek word 'cosmos' which means order or arrangement. People have been decorating their bodies for hundreds of thousands of years. It is thought that prehistoric people used ochre not only for drawing but also to colour their bodies.

Ancient **Egyptians**

The ancient Egyptians, who were very beauty conscious, had their own form of beauty parlours and the use of cosmetics was common practice. Their cosmetics were made from animal fats, olive and nut oils, seeds and flowers. Well-to-do fashionable women wore red nail polish and painted their nipples gold. So great was their consumption of cosmetics that raw materials for cosmetics became a major part of their foreign trade.

Women and men both used cosmetics and body oils. The need for skin protection and moisturisers in a hot, arid climate was perceived as necessary for both genders. Both sexes, of all classes, oiled their bodies regularly.

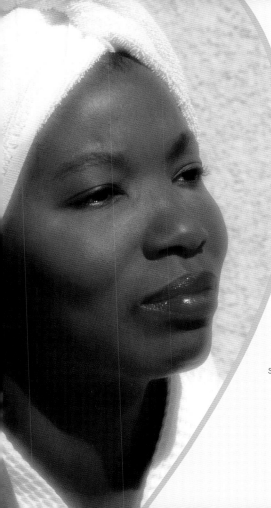

Different **cultures**

In different cultures around the world women used white powders and creams to whiten their faces, while highlighting their lips and cheeks with bright red colours. In the 1800s the fashion for Western women was pale skin with a little rouge on the cheeks to emphasise their femininity and frailty. It wasn't until the 1920s that cosmetics began to be worn by most American women on a daily basis.

Fashions have changed over the years, and keep changing year by year, with the latest trends for golden, shimmering skin and fuller lips now seen as attractive.

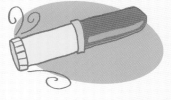

Why is facial skin
different?

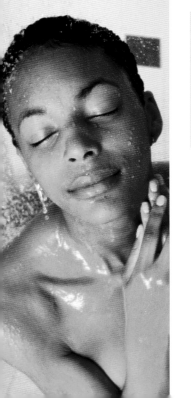

> **Skin is** the largest organ in the body, and the only one visible from the outside. Skin provides a natural barrier and protects the body from infection. It helps us retain essential fluids and regulates body temperature through sweat when it is hot and by restricting blood supply when it is cold. It also helps to remove waste products from the body and provides our sense of touch.

Facial skin

The skin on your face is the most sophisticated of all skin on the body, with many nerve endings and sebaceous glands. Facial skin is very thin and is attached to the finest muscles with the most flexibility.

Facial skin is mostly supported by a web of small muscles. Toning these muscles can give the appearance of a face-lift!

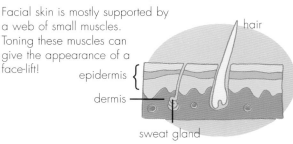

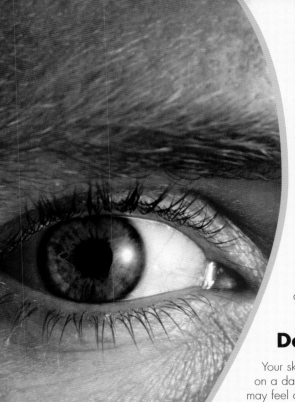

Differences in facial skin

Skin type can differ even within the face. The thickest skin is found on the forehead, jaw and chin, while the thinnest is that found on the eyelids and lips. The driest parts are the cheeks and jaw and the oiliest are on the nose, forehead and chin.

As the most expressive and exposed skin on the body, the face needs a lot of care and attention.

Daily changes

Your skin's conditions may well change on a daily basis. Some days your skin may feel dry and itchy and on others it may be oily. These changes are due to a variety of factors as you will find out later on in this book.

7

Types of **skin**

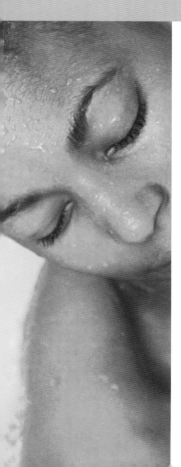

> **Skin type** is determined by how dry or oily the skin is and its pore size. Healthy, glowing skin looks radiant and youthful, whereas a dry, dull, flaky complexion can add years to your face. It is important to know what type of skin you have to give it the specific care it needs, so you can benefit from its good looks. However, any serious skin problem should be referred to a dermatologist.

Normal skin

This skin is not too oily or too dry, the skin is firm and smooth with small pores. It is naturally well moisturised.

Dry skin

Lacking natural oils, the texture of dry skin may be rough, flaky or tight. There are little or no shiny areas. The skin may have a dull appearance and become chapped if extremely dry.

Oily skin

Oily skin can make the face shiny and may have a coarse texture, especially the T-zone (forehead, nose and chin), with enlarged pores. People with oily skin may be more prone to pimples and blackheads, than other skin types.

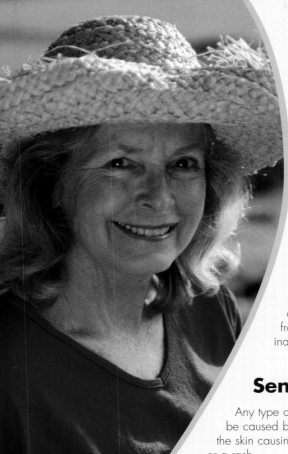

Combination skin

This is the most common skin type. In most people this means an oily T-zone (forehead, nose and chin), and normal or dry skin around the cheeks and throat.

Mature skin

This is not so much a type of skin as something that will happen to all of us. Mature skin suffers from fine lines, loss of elasticity and a loose, crepy appearance. Not always associated with age but may result from over exposure to the elements or inadequate nutrition.

Sensitive skin

Any type of skin can be sensitive. This may be caused by products that are too harsh for the skin causing irritation, reddening, stinging or a rash.

9

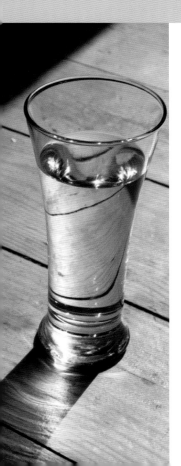

The act of living, eating, breathing and everyday wear and tear takes its toll on our skin. Although we can't stop this completely, there are measures we can take to keep our skin in optimum health and reduce the bad effects that we all hope to avoid.

Diet

The old saying, 'You are what you eat', is true. The skin reflects the body's health, and our modern lifestyle and a diet high in fats and processed food, with the resultant increase in skin problems, is testament to this.

For a great complexion and optimal skin health, just a few changes in diet can reap huge benefits. So do:

- Drink plenty of water. Around eight glasses a day, with a slice of lemon or lime, for extra flavour, will keep your skin well hydrated.

- Eat at least five servings of fruit and vegetables each day. Try to include a variety of colours. Fruit and vegetables contain antioxidants which prevent premature skin ageing.

- Eat more fish. Fatty acids found in oily fish and nuts help nourish and hydrate the skin, improving complexion.

- Include foods high in beneficial vitamins. This can have a dramatic effect on your skin.

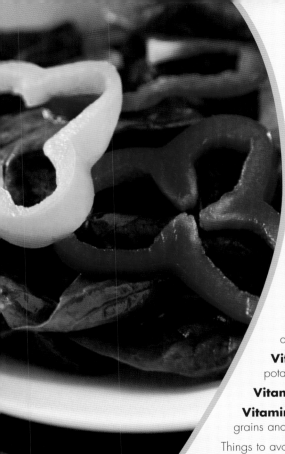

Vitamins

Vitamin A helps to prevent damage from the sun and excessive drying out. Vitamin C is needed for the production of collagen and elastin which keep the skin elastic. It also, together with vitamin E, helps to prevent skin damage from free radicals which age the skin. Vitamin E promotes healthy skin and helps reduce scarring and vitamins C and D can help with skin healing.

Some common foods containing vitamins A, C, D, and E

Vitamin A: green leafy vegetables, orange and red fruit and vegetables, eggs.

Vitamin C: citrus fruits, tomatoes, potatoes, green leafy vegetables.

Vitamin D: oily fish, milk.

Vitamin E: vegetables, nuts, seed oils, grains and wheat germ.

Things to avoid in your diet include alcohol, and snacks and fast foods that are high in fat, such as crisps, chocolate and fried foods.

11

The **environment**

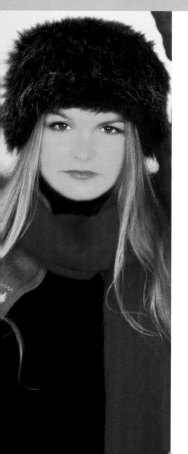

Various factors in the environment can have an adverse effect on your skin. Knowing how you can help protect yourself from the havoc they may wreak on your face will keep your skin looking healthy and glowing.

The sun

The sun can damage your skin more than any other environmental factor. Ultra-violet light from the sun damages collagen and elastin in the skin, reduces elasticity and causes wrinkling. Damage by the sun increases the risk of skin cancer. Doctors recommend wearing sunscreen or foundation with an SPF of at least 15, no matter what the weather is like.

Most skin damage occurs before the age of 18.

Using special filters on a camera, it is possible to view the damage ultra-violet rays have caused to the lower layer of your skin.

Paradoxically, sunlight is vital for the production of vitamin D. Unless certain levels of light fall upon the skin, stores of this important vitamin become depleted.

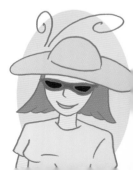

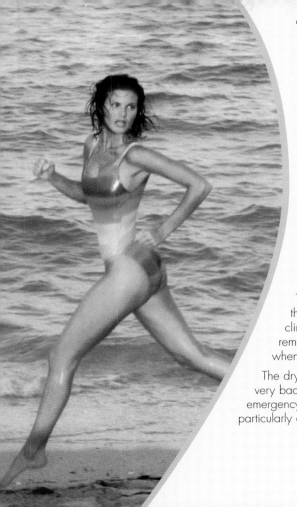

The seasons

As the seasons change, the weather presents a different set of problems for your skin.

Extremes of climate are always hard for skin to deal with, so the depths of winter and the middle of summer can be equally hard on your skin leaving it feeling rough and dehydrated. Skin responds best to humid climates, where it absorbs moisture from the air.

Dry air, heating and air conditioning draw moisture away from the skin, making it dehydrated and feeling tight.

These effects can be magnified by the shock of travelling to a different climate on holiday so it is important to remember your skin care products when you are packing.

The dry, recycled air inside aircraft is also very bad for your skin so a mid-flight emergency moisturising kit can pay dividends, particularly on long-haul flights.

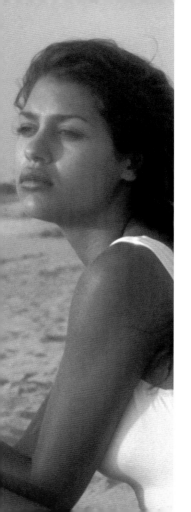

Air pollution

The world is full of air pollution which, although invisible, has drastic effects on your skin. Chemicals in the air break down the natural oils in the skin that normally keep the skin smooth and supple and can also inhibit skin repairing itself. Dirt and dust block pores in the skin and increase the number of bacteria on the face leading to spots and acne.

Smoking

Smoking has a damaging effect on the skin. Cigarette smoke and tar cause blood vessels to shrink, reducing the skin's supply of nutrients and oxygen resulting in dull, lifeless skin. It also leads to the formation of free radicals that weaken the collagen and elastin fibres in skin, leaving it prematurely wrinkled. Passive or secondary smoking is almost as bad so it always pays to keep away from smoky environments.

Gravity

You might not think about it and you certainly can't feel it, but gravity is tugging away at the skin on your face every day. Gravity is the reason that your jowls move down as you get older. While you cannot counteract the pull of gravity (yet!), regular facial massage will keep the muscles in your face trim and fit thus minimising the effects of gravity on your face.

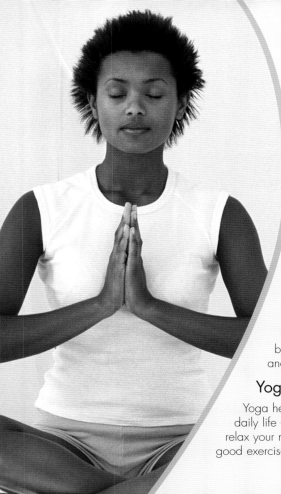

Stress

Skin problems can often be an outward sign of stress, or may just exacerbate existing problems. Possible skin reactions that may occur are acne, psoriasis, hives, itching, sweating and eczema. So be aware of the effect that stress may have on your skin. Help to combat stress by taking time out each day for relaxing or meditating. There are several ways to combat stress without resorting to medical aid including:

Exercise

Regular exercise is good for your body and is also a potent stress buster. A good workout at the gym helps to flush all the tension from your body as well as keeping you fitter and healthier.

Yoga

Yoga helps you to cope with stress in your daily life by giving you the time and space to relax your mind and body. It is also very good exercise.

15

Skin **care**

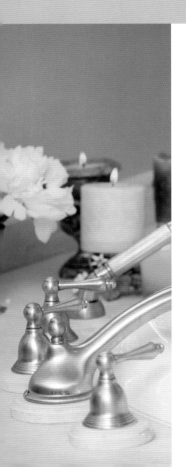

A daily skin care routine will maximise one of your most valuable assets and help you look your best. Healthy, glowing skin needs regular cleansing, moisturising and protection and requires only a few minutes of effort a day to maintain. After deciding which skin type you have, choose products that are appropriate for your skin to help with your skin care programme.

Step 1 Cleansing

Avoid using soap as it is very drying on the skin. Instead, choose a cream, lotion or gel cleanser that is gentler on the skin. First splash your face with warm water to open the pores. Apply the cleanser with cotton wool, using gentle upward strokes, then rinse with warm water. A few splashes of cold water will close the pores.

Step 2 Toning

Toning after cleansing will remove any remaining traces of make-up, stimulate circulation, close the pores and balance pH levels. Apply the toner with cotton wool, using light upward strokes.

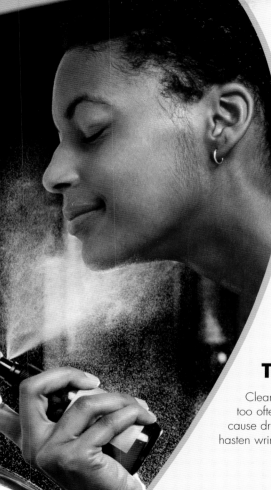

Step 3
Moisturising

Moisturisers make the skin feel softer and smoother and can plump out fine lines. All skin types need moisturising, even oily ones, and moisturiser should be applied in gentle upward strokes. It is worth considering a moisturiser that contains SPF sunscreen if you spend any time outdoors.

As important as it is to have a skin care routine, don't forget that sleep, a healthy diet and regular exercise are equally important for maintaining your skin's condition.

Tip

Cleansing the skin too often will cause dryness and hasten wrinkling.

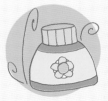

17

Common skin
problems

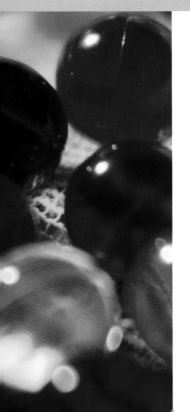

Even the best cared for skin can have problems. Most of these ailments are easily treated, but if you are unsure, consult your doctor.

Acne

Acne is most commonly suffered by people in their teens and twenties, but it can last into later life. The unsightly swellings, pustules, blackheads and tender lumps can cause embarrassment, but lots of help is available. Avoid squeezing or touching the face as this can spread infection and cause scarring. Use water-based cosmetics and remove make-up at night. A balanced diet and over-the-counter remedies are often sufficient to contain the problem, but if the acne is severe consult your doctor.

Rosacea

This is a condition that affects millions of people, manifesting in small, broken blood vessels usually on the cheeks and nose and often concurrent with acne. There is no cure, but controlling triggers such as wind, cold, heat, alcohol and stress are the main treatment. Using a high factor sunscreen every day and lowering your stress levels can also help to control the condition.

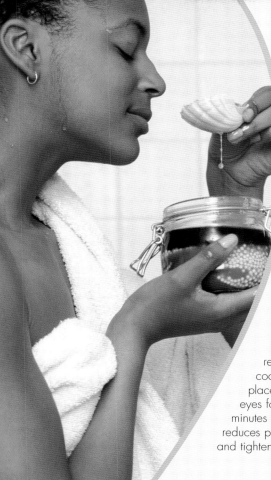

Puffy eyes

Puffy eyes afflict all of us at some time in our lives, but some people suffer more than others. Puffy eyes are caused by an accumulation of fluid in the tissues underneath the eyes. It may be linked to sinus problems or allergies.

Getting plenty of sleep and limiting your alcohol intake are good preventative measures. Limiting caffeine intake can also be beneficial.

If these suggestions don't solve the problem, lying down in a quiet room with either pieces of cucumber or cotton wool pads soaked in iced water on your eyes may help reduce the swelling. Another remedy is cooled tea-bags placed on the eyes for ten minutes which reduces puffiness and tightens the skin.

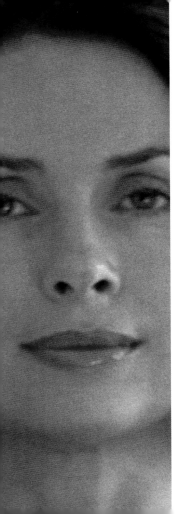

Under-eye circles

The skin under our eyes becomes thinner as we age, making the veins under the eye appear more prominent. In people with allergies the veins become swollen and more noticeable and lack of sleep accentuates the problem. Treating allergies and getting plenty of sleep are the first steps in reducing under-eye circles, as well as the cucumber and tea-bag remedies described earlier. Make-up is an excellent camouflage. Foundation and concealer applied all around the eye and blended in well will make you look as though you've just woken from a refreshing sleep.

Sensitive skin

The most common problem of sensitive skin is reaction to certain products, causing redness, irritation and blotchy skin. Treat sensitive skin and prevent adverse reactions to products by only using products that are hypoallergenic and fragrance free, as well as using the least amount of each product possible on your face. Avoid exfoliants and products containing alpha hydroxy acid and retinols which cause irritation.

Warts

Warts are very common. They are caused by viruses that normally live happily on the skin surface but penetrate the *stratum corneum* when it is damaged. Warts are most frequently seen on the fingers and the feet (when they are usually called verrucas). They can be treated by creams available from pharmacies, or by freezing.

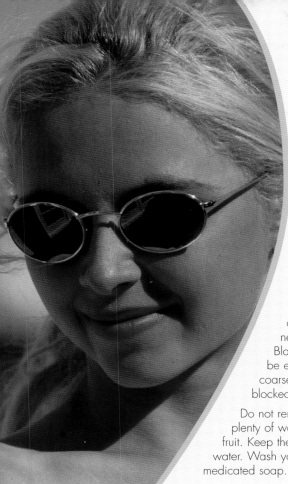

Whiteheads

These are tiny, white raised spots that are caused by the accumulation of hardened sebum or oil in the pores of the skin when sebum blocks a hair follicle deeper in the skin.

Do not remove them forcibly. Drink plenty of water and fruit juices and eat fresh fruit. Mix beauty grains and skin tonic together and rub regularly on the affected areas to dislodge the whiteheads.

Blackheads

Blackheads are not dirt and cannot be washed away. A blackhead results when dead skin cells and sebum block a hair follicle near the surface of the skin. Blackheads cause the oily skin pores to be enlarged and the texture becomes coarse and rough. When a pore is fully blocked, a pimple can result.

Do not remove blackheads forcibly. Drink plenty of water and fruit juices and eat fresh fruit. Keep the skin clean by washing it with plain water. Wash your face with warm water and a medicated soap.

21

Make-**up**

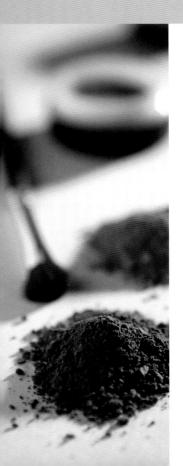

As the saying goes, 'beauty is only skin deep', but inner beauty is what makes you shine and stand out as the individual you are. Feelings of happiness and satisfaction sometimes need hard work, but finding what makes us happy in life and maintaining fulfilling relationships are more valuable than mere outer beauty.

Make-up is, however, a fantastic way of improving your general appearance and boosting your confidence, radiating your inner beauty.

What make-up to choose?

The first task is to choose make-up that suits your skin colour, skin type and eye colour. Be realistic about what suits you and, if you are unsure, get advice from a friend or beauty consultant.

Economy drive

If money is tight, consider a cheaper version of the make-up you want, many of which are excellent value for money. Some of the ingredients used in luxury brands are also used in cheaper brands!

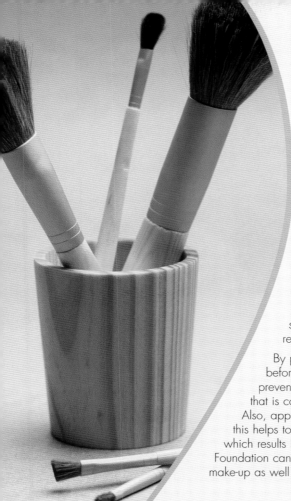

Practice makes perfect

It is important to remember that putting on make-up is not easy, and time, patience and practice are needed to create a stunning effect. If you are planning a new look for a special occasion, experiment a few days beforehand so that you can get the look you want without panicking on the day.

Making make-up last

To prevent your carefully applied make-up running, smudging or smearing, there are a few points to remember:

By patting your blusher on your lips before you apply your lipstick, you help prevent feathering and bleeding of lipstick that is commonly associated with older skin. Also, apply your lipstick with a lip brush as this helps to prevent over-application of lipstick, which results in 'kiss marks' on cups and glasses. Foundation can be used as a base for eye make-up as well as lipstick.

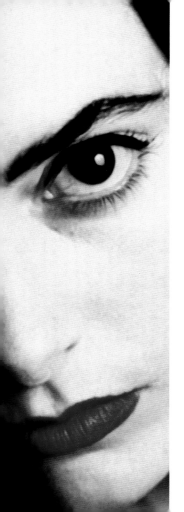

Applying your make-up

To start with, you need to cleanse, tone and moisturise your face. Use a water-based moisturiser or wait for twenty minutes after applying if your moisturiser is oily.

Foundation and concealers

These products are designed to make your skin look radiant and blemish-free. Apply a soothing or medicated ointment to pimples or inflamed areas before applying your foundation.

First apply concealer to any spots or blemishes. Choose a concealer that is slightly lighter than your skin colour. Foundation should be sheer and light to prevent cracking. Apply small amounts at a time and smooth with your fingers or a cosmetic sponge. Blend the foundation around the jawline, hairline, eyes and lips so that no lines show. The colour of your foundation should be the one that is closest to your skin colour.

Eye make-up

To neaten eyebrows pluck out any stray hairs then brush them in the direction of the hair growth. If you colour your eyebrows, match the dye to your hair colour.

Apply eyeliner to the base of your lids to shape and enhance your eyes. Adding eyeliner to the lower eyelids creates a more dramatic effect.

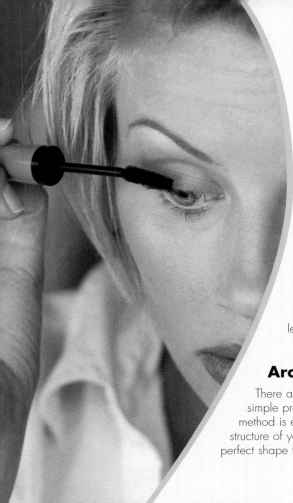

Eyeshadow comes in different forms – powder and pencil, which are suitable for all skin types, and cream, which is good for dry skin. They all come in an amazing range of colours and go on the entire lid. You can also fill in the space between your lids and eyebrows. Different colours and shades can be blended to add emphasis to the eyes.

Mascara magic

For opening the eyes and adding definition you can't beat mascara. Choose a type that suits your eyelashes, using a volumising mascara if your lashes tend to be a bit sparse, or a lengthening mascara for short lashes.

Arching your eyebrows

There are many misconceptions about this simple process. The following five-step method is easy to follow, and uses the bone structure of your face to determine what is the perfect shape for your eyebrow.

25

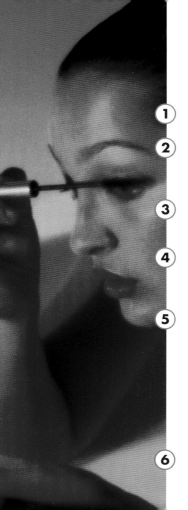

We are aiming to place the crest of the arch just to the side of your pupil, and ideally the eyebrow will curve from just inside the eye socket up to the crest.

(1) Begin by combing the brows upwards, in the direction of the hair growth.

(2) To help you during the rest of the process, colour in your brows using a brow pencil, or brow brush. If you have dark hair, use a shade lighter; if you have fair hair use a shade darker to colour.

(3) Place your pencil vertical to the edge of your nose and line it up with the inside corner of your eye. Where the pencil intersects your eyebrow is where the brow should start.

(4) To find the other end of your brow, line up the pencil, from the same edge of your nose as step 3, with the outer corner of your eye. Where your eyebrow intersects this line is the furthest point of your brow.

(5) Tweeze away any hairs that do not fall between these points.

Your eyebrows provide the overall impression of balance for your face, and therefore it's important that you ensure that your brows are level. Before you move on to the other brow, align the pencil with the outer and inner points of the brow you've shaped, and then line up the pencil with the inner corner of the other brow. Hopefully it will be in a straight line!

(6) Repeat the whole process for the other brow.

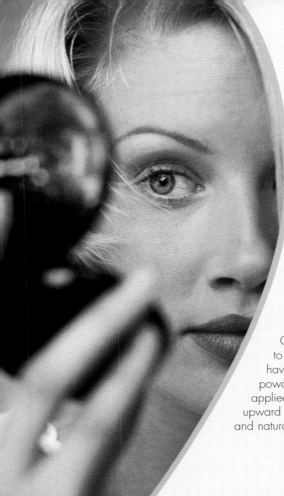

Lips and lipsticks

First line your lips with a lip liner, choosing a colour that is the same as, or slightly lighter than, your lipstick. Lipstick adheres to the lip liner, helping to keep it in place.

Try out the many different types of lipstick, from gloss to matte and cream, to see which you like best. Try mixing different shades of lipstick to create your own unique colour. To make lipstick last longer blot your lips with a tissue and then apply a second coat.

Cheeks and blusher

Choose a blush colour that is similar to the colour of your cheeks after you have exercised. Blush comes as powders or creams and should be applied sparingly. Blend gently in an upward and outward direction for a fresh and natural look.

What facials **can do**

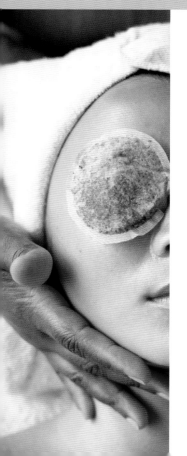

Nowadays women have a choice between salon treatments and home remedies. Both can be relaxing and effective treatments and are designed to give you natural, glowing skin.

Salon facials

Facials carried out by a beauty therapist are pampering and soothing and are performed in a relaxing atmosphere. Your skin is assessed and suitable products applied. The therapist is qualified to remove impurities such as pimples and blackheads, reducing the risk of infection and scarring.

Home facials

Facials done at home can be effective treatments for problem skins as well as a relaxing and fun way to spend half an hour. Be sure to pay close attention to cleanliness and hygiene and use only fresh ingredients to prevent introducing bacteria to your face, which can cause pimples. Be careful to avoid things that may cause a rash or irritate your skin.

Salon **facials**

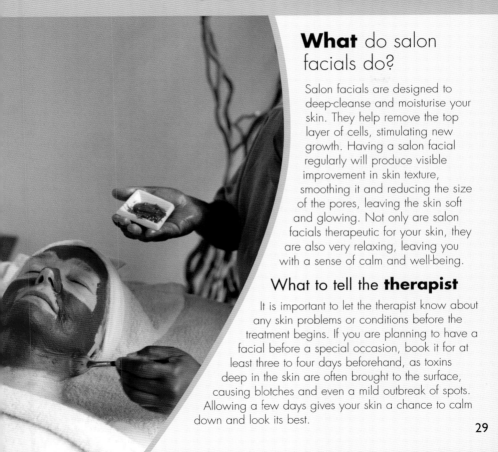

What do salon facials do?

Salon facials are designed to deep-cleanse and moisturise your skin. They help remove the top layer of cells, stimulating new growth. Having a salon facial regularly will produce visible improvement in skin texture, smoothing it and reducing the size of the pores, leaving the skin soft and glowing. Not only are salon facials therapeutic for your skin, they are also very relaxing, leaving you with a sense of calm and well-being.

What to tell the **therapist**

It is important to let the therapist know about any skin problems or conditions before the treatment begins. If you are planning to have a facial before a special occasion, book it for at least three to four days beforehand, as toxins deep in the skin are often brought to the surface, causing blotches and even a mild outbreak of spots. Allowing a few days gives your skin a chance to calm down and look its best.

29

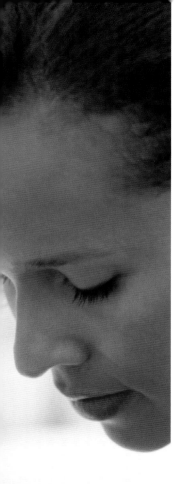

Which facial should I **choose?**

The choices of salon facials are numerous and often bewildering. Some of the most common types are described here, but if you are unsure about which to go for, discuss the options with the beauty therapist, who will be able to advise which facial is best suited to your skin.

Classic facial

This treatment includes cleansing, steaming, exfoliation, a customised face mask and moisturising. It is designed to deep-cleanse and hydrate, restoring the skin's natural beauty. It is suitable for all skin types.

Clarifying facial

For problem skins and acne, the clarifying facial cleanses and steams to remove impurities from the skin. An antibacterial mask is applied to promote healing. Oil-free moisturising soothes and calms the skin.

Exfoliating facial

A mini facial that cleanses, removes dead skin cells and moisturises, leaving the skin smooth, glowing and younger-looking. This revitalising facial is good for all skin types.

Pressure points

There are specific places on your face that can help to induce relaxation. They can also help to stimulate the skin to detoxify itself, promote circulation and rejuvenate the skin.

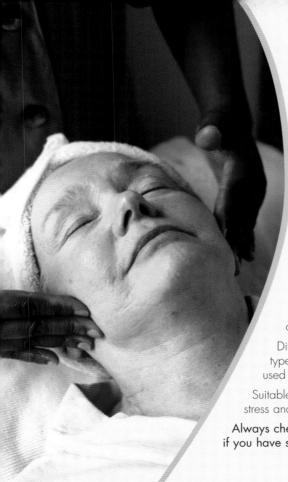

AHA facial

Known for their anti-ageing properties, AHAs (alpha-hydroxy acids) are derived from plants. This facial removes toxins and impurities and helps the skin to look smoother and healthier. It is most suitable for ageing, damaged and pigmented skins.

Aromatherapy facial

A deep-cleansing facial using selected essential oils for relaxing, detoxifying and soothing the skin and facial muscles.

Different oils are used for different types of skin, and special blends are used to treat specific issues.

Suitable for all skin types, this facial relieves stress and smooths and rejuvenates the skin.

Always check with your therapist, especially if you have sensitive skin.

31

Home **facials**

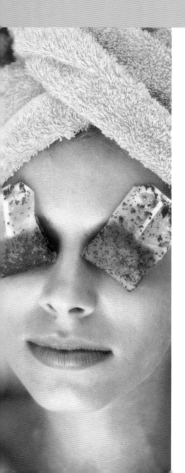

People have been using face masks for hundreds of years to improve the appearance of their skin. Today there are many different face masks to buy. However, it is easy to make your own at home using natural ingredients. That way you will know exactly what you are putting on your face!

How often should I use a face mask?

Because the ingredients in face masks are quite concentrated, they shouldn't be used more frequently than once a week. Weekly face masks are ideal, but with our hectic lifestyles this isn't always practical or possible. However, the end of winter and the end of summer are prime times to get busy with masks. Choose a mask that suits your skin type or one that targets specific skin problems. The following pages look at facials suitable for various skin types and problems, so choose one for you and start to reap the benefits.

Pamper yourself

Having some quiet time to relax while you are pampering yourself is ideal, or why not invite a friend over and have fun together?

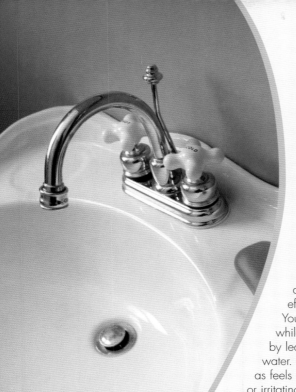

Facial steams

Steaming your face clears the
sinuses, opens your pores and
helps to relieve anxiety. It is a
good way to start your facial
and will allow the ingredients
you use in your products to
work more effectively.

Before you **steam**

Cleaning your face before
steaming removes dirt, grime
and grease and increases the
effectiveness of the procedure.
You can either steam your face
while you are sitting in the bath or
by leaning over a basin of steaming
water. Only go as close to the steam
as feels comfortable to avoid scalding
or irritating the skin. A towel draped
over your head will form a tent, trapping
the steam. Stay under for as long as you
feel comfortable.

Face **masks**

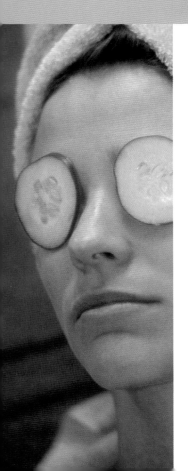

Face masks improve skin elasticity, tone and texture and stimulate cell renewal. Choose from a variety of ingredients to nourish and replenish your skin and reveal a radiant new you. Many of the ingredients will already be in your kitchen cupboard, and all you need is a fork, spoon and mixing bowl. You may want to blend the ingredients in a food processor for a smoother mixture, but blending by hand will be almost as effective.

Remember to use the freshest ingredients possible for maximum effect – it is possible to use only organic products if you prefer. The advantage of using fresh products is that they don't contain any preservatives or additives.

Hygiene

When making your own masks, remember that hygiene is essential. To begin, wash your hands with soap and water, then wash all equipment that you will be using. Make sure all working surfaces are spotlessly clean.

You may find it useful to have a supply of clean, old towels and face cloths, as well as a headband to keep your hair clean and out of the way.

The following recipes will help you achieve smooth, glowing skin, so get mixing and enjoy the benefits!

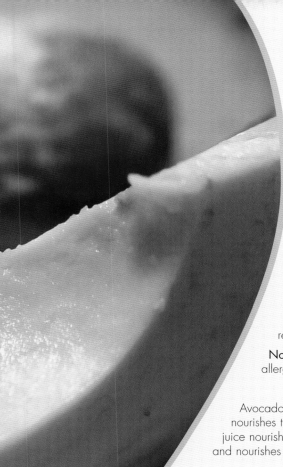

Nourishing mask for **dry** skin

Ingredients:

50 g avocado

2 tbsp fresh orange juice

1 tsp honey

3 or 4 drops chamomile essential oil

Mash the avocado, then add the remaining ingredients and mix together. If the mixture is too thick add more orange juice. Spread the mask over your face and neck and leave for at least 30 minutes. Rinse off with warm water. Any remaining mixture will keep for 1–2 days in the refrigerator.

Note: do not use if you suffer from an allergy to citrus fruits.

Avocado is rich in vitamins and minerals and nourishes the skin. The vitamin C in orange juice nourishes the skin. Honey is rich in minerals and nourishes and softens.

35

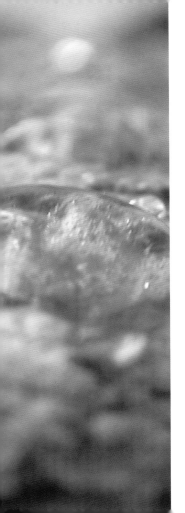

Soothing mask for **sensitive** or irritated skin

Ingredients:

1 small pot natural yogurt with live cultures

2 tsp honey

2 tbsp oatmeal

Blend ingredients together. Apply a thin layer to your face and neck with fingers and leave for a minimum of twenty minutes. Wash skin with warm water to remove mask and pat skin dry.

Oatmeal softens and soothes the skin. Honey acts as an anti-inflammatory and is rich in vitamins and minerals, stimulating skin healing and regeneration.

Tip

Yogurt, eaten, used to wash the hair or as a face mask, improves your hair and your skin.

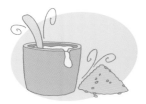

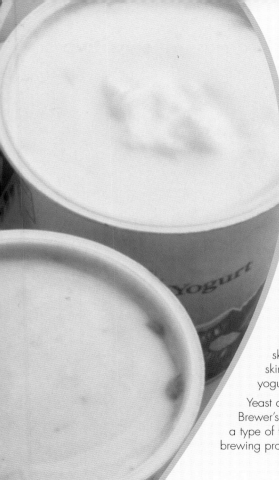

Cleansing mask for
oily skin

Ingredients:

3 tbsp natural yogurt with
live cultures

1 tsp Brewer's yeast

Mix the ingredients together to
form a thin paste. Apply it to
the oily areas and leave for
15–20 minutes. Rinse with
warm water, then splash face
with cold water to close pores.
Pat skin dry.

Yogurt softens and has a mild
bleaching effect on the skin. Its
enzymes stimulate cell activity in the
skin and restore the pH balance of the
skin, which feels as soft as silk after the
yogurt is washed away.

Yeast deep cleans and tightens pores.
Brewer's yeast is the dried, pulverised cells of
a type of fungus, which is a by-product of the
brewing process.

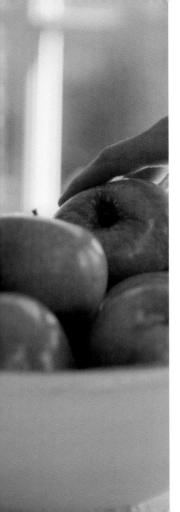

Exfoliating mask for all skin types

Ingredients:

1 tbsp oatmeal

2 tbsp natural yogurt with live cultures

¼ apple, grated

Mix the oatmeal and yogurt to form a paste. Add the apple and blend the ingredients together well.

Apply to the skin and leave for twenty minutes, then rinse with warm water. Pat the skin dry.

Oatmeal soothes irritated skin and acts as a mild exfoliant; yogurt has a softening and bleaching effect on the skin; apple cleans and acts as a gentle exfoliant.

Tip

Exfoliating encourages the skin to renew itself at a faster rate, and brings new skin cells to the skin surface for a fresh-faced look.

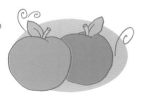

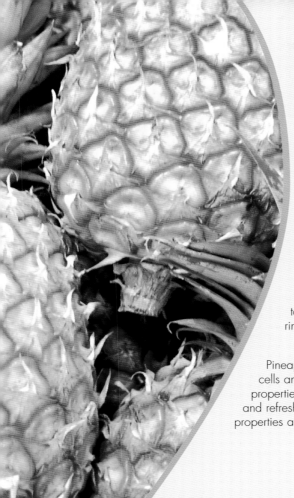

Reviving mask for the treatment of **dull** skin

Ingredients:

1 thick slice fresh pineapple

2 tbsp honey

Mash, or purée, the pineapple. Add the honey and mix together to form a smooth consistency. Spread the mixture onto your face and pat with the fingertips until the honey feels tacky. Leave for twenty minutes then rinse with warm water.

Pineapple helps rid the skin of dead skin cells and dirt and has anti-inflammatory properties. It also acts as a mild astringent and refresher. Honey has antibacterial properties and softens the skin.

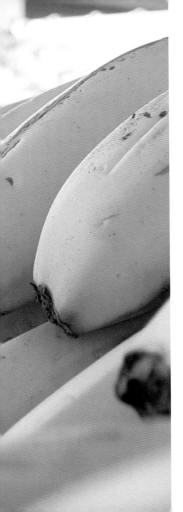

Banana and honey mask for **dry** and **sensitive** skins

Ingredients:

½ banana

2 tsp honey

1 egg

1 tbsp oatmeal

Mash the banana. Add the other ingredients and mix together until they form a thick paste. Spread the mixture on your face and leave for 15–20 minutes. Rinse with warm water and pat the skin dry.

Bananas are rich in minerals and vitamins and nourish the skin; honey acts as an anti-inflammatory and has skin-softening properties; egg nourishes and tightens the skin; oatmeal soothes and softens the skin.

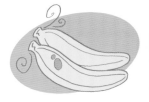

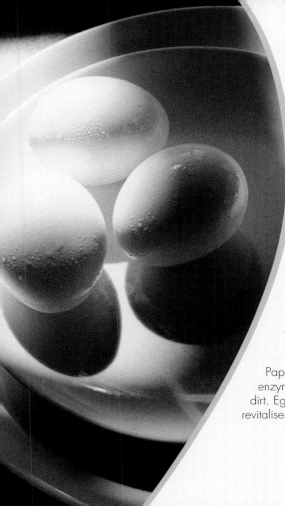

Egg and papaya mask for cleansing and revitalising **tired** skin

Ingredients:

½ papaya

1 egg white

Remove the seeds and mash the papaya. Blend it with the egg white until it has a smooth consistency. Spread the mixture over your face and leave for twenty minutes. Rinse with warm water. Pat the skin dry.

Papaya contains papain, an enzyme that helps remove dead cells and dirt. Egg white tightens pores and revitalises the skin.

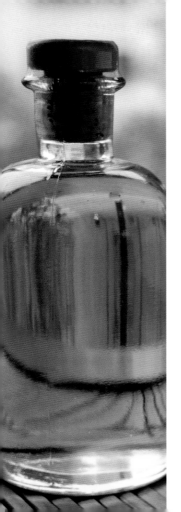

A honey and olive oil mask to **nourish** and **soften** mature skin

Ingredients:

2 tbsp honey

2 tsp olive oil

Mix the honey and olive oil together. Apply the mixture to your face and pat until the mask feels tacky. Leave for twenty minutes, then rinse with warm water. Pat the skin dry.

Honey is rich in minerals which stimulate skin regeneration. It also has mild antibiotic properties which will help to keep your skin healthy. Manuka honey is especially rich in these properties. Olive oil soothes and moisturises the skin.

Tip

As we get older, our skin becomes drier. Moisturising becomes more important, as does protection against sun damage.

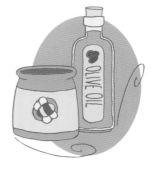

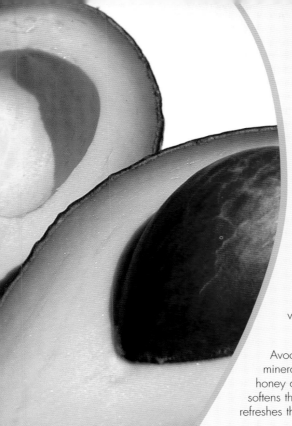

A **softening** and **refreshing** mask for all skin types

Ingredients:

½ avocado

2 tsp honey

1 tbsp natural yogurt with live cultures

Mash the avocado, then add the other ingredients and mix together until they form a smooth, creamy consistency. Apply to the skin and leave for 10–15 minutes. Rinse with warm water and pat skin dry.

Avocado is rich in vitamins and minerals and nourishes the skin; honey acts as an anti-inflammatory and softens the skin; yogurt softens and refreshes the skin.

Natural facial **toner**

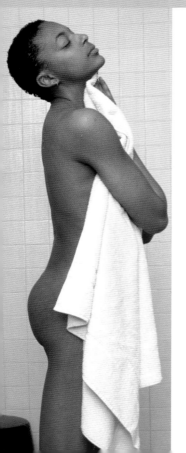

> **After cleansing** and applying a face mask, you could follow up with a home-made toner that nourishes and protects the skin. Toners can help to restore the natural pH of the skin and moisturise and condition, enhancing the soothed and refreshed feeling.

Use distilled water for purity, adding essential oils for a gentle tone. Make up the toner and store it in a clean bottle. A glass spray bottle is useful, but you can also apply toner with a cotton wool pad. Store in a cool place.

Chamomile toner for **normal/dry** skins

Ingredients:

200 ml distilled water

10 drops rose oil

7 drops chamomile oil

Mix all the ingredients together; pour into a clean bottle and shake well before each use.

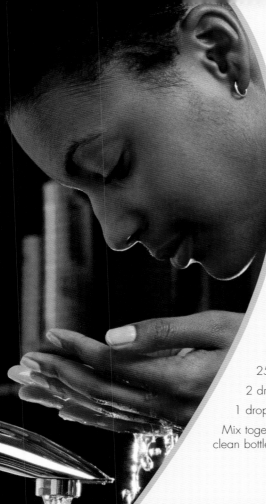

Tea tree toner for **oily** skins

Ingredients:

100 ml chamomile tea made with distilled water

100 ml witch hazel

10 drops tea tree oil

Mix all the ingredients together well; pour into a clean bottle and shake before use.

A refreshing **peppermint** and clary sage toner

Ingredients:

250 ml distilled water

2 drops peppermint oil

1 drop clary sage oil

Mix together all the ingredients; pour into a clean bottle and shake well before each use.

Natural **moisturisers**

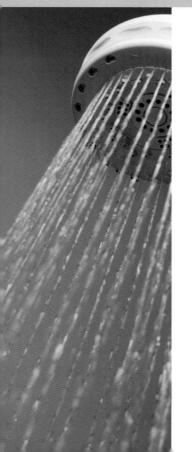

> **You can** enjoy the freshness of a home-made moisturiser, mixing up a skin-quenching lotion for soft, supple skin. These are ideal if you are allergic to preservatives and fragrances. Remember to wash your hands before preparing and applying your moisturiser.

Honey and milk moisturiser for **smooth,** baby-soft skin

Ingredients:

100 ml dried chamomile

100 ml milk

2 tbsp honey

1 tbsp wheat germ

Soak the chamomile in the milk for 3–4 hours. Strain the mixture, keeping the liquid. Add the honey and wheat germ to the liquid and blend well. Pour the mixture into a bottle. This moisturiser will keep for up to one week in the refrigerator.